Table of Contents

What are the symptoms of obesity?

General symptoms of obesity include weight gain, needing to buy progressively larger-sized clothing, and a change in the shape of your body due to the accumulation of excessive fat. In men, excessive fat stores tend to accumulate in the waist. In women, extra fat is often stored in the hips and thighs. However, in both sexes, extra fat can accumulate throughout the body, including such areas as the face, neck, feet and hands.

Body mass index and other measures

A medical sign of obesity or overweight is having a higher than normal body mass index (BMI). BMI is one method used by healthcare professionals to calculate an estimate of the amount of body fat you are carrying. BMI is accurate for most people, but may not be an accurate indicator of excessive fat stores for certain populations.

For example, if you are an athlete with developed muscles, which weigh more than fat, you may have a healthy level of body fat but still rank as overweight on the BMI. Also, BMI is not accurate in determining fat stores in pregnant women and people with diseases that cause moderate to large amounts of water retention.

While a high BMI identifies potential weight issues, it is not enough to diagnose obesity and will not indicate any specific health risks. To better determine the risk of developing weight-related health problems, other indicators are assessed by healthcare providers. These include:

Obesity-related diseases and conditions, such as high blood pressure or a sedentary lifestyle, and other factors

Waist size, as excessive fat in the waistline is associated with an increased risk for obesity-related diseases, such as diabetes

What causes obesity?

Obesity is caused by consuming more calories than necessary to fuel your body's activity level and metabolic processes in a given time period. Extra calories are stored as fat if there is not a corresponding increase in activity to burn calories.

Primary causes of an increase in stored body fat include:

- Diets that are high in calories, fat and sugar
- Sedentary lifestyle without sufficient exercise

Less often, obesity may be directly or indirectly caused by certain untreated diseases or conditions including:

- Certain medications, such as corticosteroids, antidepressants, and seizure medications

- Cushing syndrome (overproduction of the hormone cortisol)

- Hypothyroidism (underactive thyroid)

- Polycystic ovarian syndrome (PCOS, which produces high levels of certain hormones)

Is obesity genetic?

Although researchers have identified several genes that appear to be associated with obesity, most believe that one single gene is not responsible for the entire obesity epidemic.

However, studies have shown that a predisposition toward obesity can be inherited. Studies of identical twins, including those who have been raised separately, have estimated that inheritability of obesity can be as high as 77%. In rare cases, genetic defects in children can affect production of hormones related to appetite stimulation, such as leptin, which can result in severe obesity.

Scientists also have proposed a "thrifty genotype" hypothesis based on our ancestors' lack of regular access to food. This theory suggests that the human body is "trained" to retain weight rather than lose it, which can make it difficult to maintain a healthy weight in environments where food—and high-calorie food, at that—is readily available.

Along with genetics, lifestyle factors within families play a role in obesity, as children are more likely to model eating or exercise habits from those of the people around them.

What are the risk factors for obesity?

There are many factors that may encourage, influence or contribute to the development of obesity. These factors may occur alone or may be linked with other factors, such as aging in combination with a sedentary lifestyle.

Factors that can increase the risk of obesity include:

- Aging, which slows metabolism and the rate at which you burn calories
- Cultural factors, such as overeating or eating high-calorie foods as a part of certain cultural practices or gatherings
- Eating a diet that is high in calories, fat and sugar. Your caloric intake may be influenced by the easy accessibility of super-sized, high-calorie foods, which also tend to be less

expensive and more convenient than healthier foods.

- Family history of obesity. Obesity tends to run in families, which may be linked to both genetics and the development of similar dietary and exercise habits.

- Insomnia or poor sleep habits

- Menopause

- Pregnancy

- Poor socioeconomic status. People from low-income backgrounds have a greater risk for obesity.

- Sedentary lifestyle

- Smoking cessation. Some people who quit smoking gain weight. After quitting smoking, the sense of taste and smell improves, which may encourage some people to overeat.

- Stress, depression, anxiety, and other mental and emotional disturbances

- Weight gain during pregnancy that is not lost after giving birth
- Working night shifts or odd shifts and getting poor-quality sleep

There is a strong relationship between economic status and obesity, especially among women. Women who are poor and of lower social status are more likely to be obese than women of higher socioeconomic status. The occurrence of obesity is also highest among minority groups, especially among women.

Overeating, along with a sedentary lifestyle, contributes to obesity. These are lifestyle choices that can be affected by behavior change. Eating a diet in which a high percentage of calories come from sugary, high-fat, refined foods promotes weight gain. Lack of regular exercise contributes to obesity in adults and makes it difficult to maintain weight loss. In children, inactivity, such as watching television, playing too many video games, or sitting at a computer, contributes to obesity.

Reducing your risk of obesity

You may be able to lower your risk of obesity and its complications by:

- Eating a healthy diet focusing on low-calorie, high-nutrient foods, including lean meats, fruits, vegetables and whole grains. Avoid processed foods high in saturated fats, and limit alcohol and sweets to occasional treats.
- Exercising regularly, ideally 150 to 300 minutes per week of moderate-intensity activity, such as tennis, biking, dancing, gardening, swimming or brisk walking
- Finding weight-loss support through friends or online groups, to help stay motivated and keep yourself accountable
- Getting quality sleep, ideally 7 to 8 hours each night. Sleep deprivation can cause increased

appetite, and loss of sleep can make losing weight more difficult. Conversely, conditions caused by obesity, such as sleep apnea, can result in poor sleep.

- Lowering stress through activities, such as meditation and mindfulness. Stress hormones, such as cortisol, can cause weight gain. Feelings of stress can also lead to overeating, particularly of comfort foods that are high in fat and sugar.

- Monitoring your weight to be aware of your progress and to identify weight gain patterns based on your diet and activity

- Losing 1 to 2 pounds a week is considered a healthy rate of weight loss. Avoid weight-loss fads or "crash" diets that can be unhealthy and are not sustainable. For some people, intermittent fasting can be an effective tool for managing diet when done properly. Your doctor can work with you to establish weight loss goals and guide you toward resources and support to help you achieve them.

What are the diet and nutrition tips for obesity?

Healthy eating habits are essential to addressing obesity and to achieving and maintaining a healthy weight. By working with your doctor and possibly a nutritionist, you can determine your target daily calorie intake and build a nutrition plan that meets your weight loss goals.

A nutritious diet includes not just what you eat, but also how much and when you eat. Tips for diet and nutrition with a goal of weight loss or healthy weight maintenance include:

- Avoiding processed foods, such as fast food, potato chips, packaged cookies, and frozen pizza

- Cooking meals yourself, to help control ingredients and manage portions

- Drinking plenty of water, while avoiding high-sugar beverages, such as regular soda, sweetened tea, or fruit juice. Be wary of sports drinks, too, as they include high amounts of sugar.

- Eating a healthy breakfast every morning to avoid overeating later in the day

- Focusing on whole foods that are minimally processed, including whole grains, colorful vegetables, whole fruits, lean fish and poultry, nuts and seeds, and plant oils, such as olive oil

- Keeping a food journal to monitor your eating habits and make changes where necessary. Even if you don't track every calorie, it helps to have an awareness of what—and how much—you are eating each day.

- Limiting alcohol, which contains "empty" calories and can make you more likely to overeat

- Limiting refined grains and sugars, including white bread, white pasta, and white rice

- Reducing red meat in favor of lean poultry or fish. Cut back on cold cuts too, which add sodium and preservatives. A piece of fresh roasted turkey is healthier than packaged turkey from the deli.

- Slowing down and eating smaller portions, to give your body time to tell you when it's had enough food. This can also help improve mindful eating, which allows you to focus on making good choices and savor the food in front of you.

How do doctors diagnose obesity?

Your doctor likely measures your weight at each of your appointments. If your weight increases significantly over time, he or she may discuss factors that could be contributing to your weight gain.

The most common screening tool for overweight and obesity is body mass index (BMI). Doctors calculate this measure using a formula based on your weight and height. In adults, a BMI from 18.5 to 24.9 is considered normal while a BMI of more than 25 is considered overweight. A person is considered obese if the BMI is greater than 30 and morbidly obese if the BMI is 40 or greater. When assessing a child's weight, the BMI is calculated and then plotted on a BMI for age percentile curve.

It's important to note that a high BMI does not necessarily mean someone's weight is unhealthy. For example, some people may have a lot of muscle, which is denser than fat. This means they have a higher weight, and thus a higher BMI, but their body fat remains low.

Another measure of obesity is the waist-to-hip ratio (WHR). The WHR is a measurement tool that looks at the proportion of fat stored on the waist, and hips and buttocks. The waist circumference indicates abdominal fat. A waist circumference more than 40 inches in men and more than 35 inches in women may increase the risk of heart disease and other diseases associated with being overweight.

What are the treatments for obesity?

In most cases, obesity in adults and children results from consuming too many calories and not getting enough physical activity. Treatment of obesity includes developing and following a sensible, comprehensive lifelong plan to reduce your caloric intake while ensuring good nutrition and hydration, and increasing physical activity.

Effective weight loss plans often incorporate some form of support through a medically approved weight loss group or organization, such as Weight Watchers. Counseling may also be recommended to help you change certain behaviors or address issues that lead you to overeat, such as anxiety and depression.

In general, experts advise that you lose no more than 1 to 2 pounds a week to achieve a safe, healthy weight loss that can be maintained. Recommended calorie intake and exercise levels will vary among individuals, depending on age, sex, general fitness level, medical history, and other factors. Very low-calorie diets or diets that are not well-balanced are generally not recommended because they can lead to rebound weight gain, poor nutrition, and other health problems.

Consult with your healthcare provider before starting any weight reduction plan so he or she can monitor health conditions, such as blood pressure and blood sugar levels, and help you develop the most effective, safe and healthy weight-loss plan for you. Your provider or weight loss support group will help set you up for success with realistic expectations in the days, weeks and months ahead.

Medications used to treat obesity

When a comprehensive diet and exercise program is not enough to help a severely obese person lose weight, medications or surgery may be an option to help treat obesity. '

You should not take any weight-reduction medications, supplements, or herbal preparations without first consulting with your physician or healthcare provider. Over-the-counter (OTC) products may cause serious side effects or interactions with the medications you take and many have not been tested by the Food and Drug Administration (FDA) to prove they are safe or effective.

The FDA has approved these weight loss medications:

- Contrave is the brand name for a combination of bupropion (an antidepressant that can decrease appetite) and naltrexone (an anti-addiction drug that can also suppress hunger). People who take or have taken opioid medications, or those in recovery from alcohol or drug addiction, should avoid Contrave.

- Orlistat, sold under the brand names Alli (60 mg dose, OTC) and Xenical (120 mg dose, prescription), is a medication that reduces the absorption of fats; fat calories; and vitamins A, D, E and K by the body. Rare cases of liver injury or liver failure have been reported with both forms of orlistat.

- Qsymia is the brand name for an extended-release combination of phentermine (an appetite suppressant) and topiramate (an antiepileptic drug that has a side effect of weight loss). Women who are or may become pregnant should avoid Qsymia, as it can increase the risk of birth defects. Qsymia may also interact with certain MAOI (monoamine oxidase inhibitor) antidepressants.

Surgical procedures used to treat obesity

Weight loss surgery, or bariatric surgery, may help some seriously obese people who have not lost weight by attempting lifestyle and dietary changes, or who have serious complications of obesity, such as type 2 diabetes or cardiovascular disease. Typically, these procedures target the gastrointestinal (GI) tract, reducing the amount of absorbable nutrients.

The most common surgical methods include:

- Gastric band, or Lap-Band, involves placing a band around the upper portion of the stomach to make a smaller pouch for food, which limits how much food you can eat and makes you feel full sooner.

- Roux-en-Y gastric bypass involves creating a small stomach pouch with a bypass around part of the small intestine, which is where most calories are absorbed.

- Sleeve gastrectomy, also known as vertical sleeve gastrectomy, removes about 80% of the stomach, restricting the amount of food you can consume. This procedure is for people with severe obesity (a BMI of 40 or higher) and in rare cases is paired with an intestinal bypass that limits the absorption of proteins and fats.

What are the potential complications of obesity?

Complications of obesity can be serious, even life-threatening. You can treat obesity and minimize the risk of complications by following the treatment plan you and your healthcare professional design specifically for you.

Potential complications of obesity include:

- Cancer including prostate, rectum, colon, ovaries, uterus, cervix and breast
- Cardiovascular conditions, such as heart disease, high cholesterol, heart failure, high blood pressure, and stroke
- Depression and other mental and emotional issues
- Disability

- Gallbladder disease

- Gout

- Gynecologic problems, such as infertility and irregular periods

- Hyperlipidemia

- Metabolic syndrome

- Nonalcoholic fatty liver disease

- Osteoarthritis

- Skin problems, such as impaired wound healing

- Sleep apnea, resulting in hypoxemia (low levels of oxygen in the blood)

- Thromboembolism

- Type 2 diabetes

1. Type 2 Diabetes

Type 2 diabetes is a common health problem. It occurs when your blood sugar levels are too high. About 4 in 5 (80%) people with type 2 diabetes are obese or overweight. Extra fat tissue may change the way your body is able to use blood sugar, experts believe.

2. Osteoarthritis

Your bones have a protective covering—called cartilage—where they rub together at your joints. Osteoarthritis happens when this protection wears away, causing joint pain and stiffness. Extra pounds can cause osteoarthritis by putting extra pressure on joints, which wears down this protective layer.

3. Cancer

Obesity is linked to a higher risk for certain types of cancer. Breast, colon, kidney, pancreatic and thyroid cancers are all more common in obese people. Why? Fat cells produce hormones, and it's possible that some of these hormones may contribute to cancer.

4. Sleep Apnea

In this common sleep disorder, your breathing stops several times during the night. Sleep apnea can make you feel very tired during the day and increase your risk for health problems, such as diabetes. Obesity is the #1 risk factor for developing sleep apnea. Obese people may be more prone to the problem because of extra fatty tissue around the upper airway. This may make the airway smaller and more likely to close up.

5. Stroke

A stroke occurs when blood flow to a part of the brain is blocked. And the effects of a stroke can be devastating. About half of stroke survivors have trouble with mobility. Some strokes are fatal. High blood pressure—which is common with obesity—is a strong risk factor for strokes.

6. High Blood Pressure

Obesity can raise your blood pressure. When your body is large, your heart has to work harder to pump blood through it. This increases the pressure in your arteries and veins. High blood pressure can damage your heart and lead to heart disease.

7. Heart Disease

Heart disease is a term that describes a number of heart problems, including heart attack, heart failure, and heart valve problems. Heart problems are the number one cause of death in the United States. Obesity increases your risk for problems that may contribute to heart disease, such as high cholesterol.

8. High Cholesterol

People who are overweight or obese tend to have higher levels of triglycerides and LDL—or "bad"—cholesterol. They also tend to have lower levels of HDL—or "good"—cholesterol. These cholesterol and triglyceride levels increase your risk for heart disease.

9. Pregnancy-Related Problems

Being overweight or obese during pregnancy can affect both the baby and the mother. For example, obese pregnant women are at risk of developing gestational diabetes and high blood pressure during pregnancy. Both can cause complications for mom and baby. A premature birth is also more likely if the mother is obese.

10. Kidney Disease

Obesity increases your risk of the two health problems most likely to cause kidney disease— high blood pressure and diabetes. Kidney disease causes waste to build up in your body. You may need dialysis or a transplant if the disease worsens to the point of kidney failure.

Home Remedies For Obesity: Procedure, Recovery, Risk & Complication

Obesity is the number one reason for many illnesses that hamper your health. In simple terms, it is an excessive accumulation of fat in the body which is not good for your lifestyle and health. They also make you susceptible to several other health problems. There are many effective ways to curb obesity and some of them can include home remedies like the one listed below.

Lemon Juice:

Lemon juice can be described as the best home remedy for fighting obesity. It improves digestion and also aids in the detoxification of the body. It is one of the finest fat-burning mechanisms if used regularly.

To use this, mix 2 teaspoons of fresh lemon juice, a teaspoon of honey, and one-half teaspoon of black pepper powder in one glass of water. Mix well and drink it on an empty stomach. You can use this regularly until you see visible results.

Green Tea:

Green tea is another remedy that is gaining in popularity to promote weight loss. It slows down your weight gain and burns fat to a vast extent thus curbing obesity. You can try out natural green teas available in the market mixing it with honey. You can even add a dash of ginger to it for the best results. You can safely have green tea three or four times a day.

Cayenne Pepper:

Cayenne pepper helps in controlling obesity and also aids in weight loss. It contains a special property that rouses your body to burn more fat. It also improves digestion drastically. You can use this by mixing cayenne pepper with a glass of water. Mix a dash of lemon juice to it. Stir well and drink it regularly for a month. You can see visible changes soon.

Drink water:

As per the researcher, drinking water can help you to burn more calories. When you take water before meals it also decreases your calorie intake. Water is most effective when compared to other beverages for weight loss.

Aloe vera:

As per the researcher aloe vera promotes the burning of calories. It also helps in the breakdown of fat. You can take aloe vera in the form of juice.

Ginger:

Ginger contains a compound called gingerol which helps in the breakdown of fat into energy.

Basil leaves:

Basil leaves contain a certain compound that reduces the blood cholesterol level and results in weight loss.

Fibre-rich diet:

Adding fibre rich food to your diet gives you the feeling of fullness especially when it's water-soluble fibre. It also helps reduce the feeling of an empty stomach fre🞐uently.

Proper sleep:

As per the studies conducted by researchers it has been observed that people who don't get enough sleep are more likely to gain weight. Proper sleep leads to the regulation of hormones necessary for metabolism.

Green vegetable:

Green vegetables contain large amounts of nutrients, fibre, and water that prevent weight gain.

Obesity can be reduced by taking green vegetables, basil leaves, aloe vera juice, fiber-rich diet, ginger,

green tea, lemon juice, green tea. Take proper sleep
and stay hydrated.

Are there any side effects of remedies for obesity?

Safe and completely herbal, these remedies show no side effects. Just make sure that you buy from trusted stores and reputed brands.

Try brewing green tea leaves rather than tea bags, as they are more effective in fighting extra fat.

Do not use cayenne pepper in high quantities as it might be too hot for you. Commonly, lemon juice is good for health.

However, if you see no significant change in your body even after a month, give it a rest as your acidity levels will go up otherwise.

If you are unsure about any of these remedies, consult your doctor for advice. This is especially important if you suffer from high blood pressure or gastric problems.

Despite being effective, certain home remedies have some side effects which vary from person to person, so choose your home remedy only if you are not allergic or sensitive to the particular substance. Do not use any home remedies in excess as it may be harmful to health.

What are the post-remedy guidelines?

To get in shape, you must avoid eating fatty and oily foods apart from following these home remedies.

Have lots of water to keep yourself hydrated throughout the day. It will flush out toxins efficiently too.

Don't go for over the counter products for losing weight, as these are either ineffective or harmful.

Exercise regularly and stick to the diet laid down by the dietician.

Eat 5 to 6 small meals instead of 3 large meals, as this will improve your metabolism and digestion.

Remember it is not only the exercise that makes you lose fat but also a strict diet regime.

Follow the guidelines. Avoid eating oily foods, junk foods. Stay hydrated. Exercise regularly. Follow a proper diet. Eat small frequent meals.

How long does it take to recover or to get rid of obesity?

The more obese you are, the more time it will take you to get in shape and to reach a healthy weight. You will have to maintain healthy eating habits throughout your life and exercise at least 4 or 5 days a week, even if it is for half an hour. Avoid junk food as much as you can and consume more fresh fruits and vegetables. Cut back on alcohol as well. Try to drink 6 to 8 glasses of water every day and think positive.

The time of recovery from obesity depends on how much obese you are. If you are more obese it will take more time to get you into shape.

Are the results of the home remedies for obesity are permanent?

Since obesity very much depends on your lifestyle and eating habits, the results cannot be permanent. If you go back to oily food after following a healthy diet for a while, you will gain back the weight you lost previously. Instead, develop a love for fresh fruits and veggies, lean meat and wholewheat rice and pieces of bread. Try avoiding OTC medications for reducing weight as they cause more damage than good in the long run.

There are many reasons due to which weight gain can occur. Hence have yourself evaluated by a dietician and your doctor to seek out the best diet plan to stay fit. Also, exercise regularly to shed those extra kilos and to stay active.

No, the results are not permanent if a healthy lifestyle is not maintained. You can again gain weight if you don't eat a healthy diet. Follow the diet plan given by your dietician or doctor.

Is there any training or experts required to perform these natural remedies for obesity?

These home remedies are safe and no training is required to follow them. However, you must know the exact cause of your obesity and try to rectify it accordingly. Often, having healthy home-cooked food and exercising regularly can help. Sometimes, obesity may not be just about eating unhealthy foods. Visit your physician if you do not find any difference in your weight after following these treatments.

No, there is no need for training or expert assistance since these home remedies are easy to perform. But if after following the remedies you are not seeing any improvement then it's recommended to visit your doctor.

Diet

Obesity can be prevented by following basic principles of healthy eating. Here are simple changes you can make to your eating habits that will help you lose weight and prevent obesity.

Eat five a day: Focus on eating at least five to seven servings of whole fruits and vegetables every day. Fruits and vegetables constitute low-calorie foods. According to WHO, there is convincing evidence that eating fruits and vegetables decreases the risk of obesity.2 They contain higher amounts of nutrients and are associated with a lower risk for diabetes and insulin resistance. Their fiber content in particular helps you feel full with fewer calories, helping to prevent weight gain.

Avoid processed foods: Highly processed foods, like white bread and many boxed snack foods, are a common source of empty calories, which tend to add up quickly. A 2019 study found that subjects who were offered a highly processed diet consumed more calories and gained weight, while those offered a minimally processed diet ate less and lost weight.[3]

Reduce sugar consumption: It is important to keep your intake of added sugars low. The American Heart Association recommends that the intake of added sugar not exceed six teaspoons daily for women and nine teaspoons daily for men.[4] Major sources of added sugar to avoid include sugary beverages, including sodas and energy or sports drinks; grain desserts like pies, cookies, and cakes; fruit drinks (which are seldom 100% fruit juice); candy; and dairy desserts like ice cream.

Limit artificial sweeteners: Artificial sweeteners have been linked to obesity and diabetes. If you feel you must use a sweetener, opt for a small amount of honey, which is a natural alternative.

Skip saturated fats: A 2018 study shows that eating foods high in saturated fat contributes to obesity.5 Focus instead on sources of healthy fats (monounsaturated and polyunsaturated fats) like avocados, olive oil, and tree nuts. Even healthy fats are recommended to be limited to 20% to 35% of daily calories, and people with elevated cholesterol or vascular disease may need an even lower level.

Sip wisely: Drink more water and eliminate all sugared beverages from your diet. Make water your go-to beverage; unsweetened tea and coffee are fine, too. Avoid energy drinks and sports drinks, which not only contain an overwhelming amount of added sugar, but have been shown (in the case of the former) to pose potential dangers to the cardiovascular system.

Cook at home: Studies looking at the freuency of home meal preparation have found that both men and women who prepared meals at home were less likely to gain weight. They were also less likely to develop type 2 diabetes.6

Try a plant-based diet: Eating a plant-based diet has been associated with greater overall health and much lower rates of obesity. To achieve this, fill your plate with whole vegetables and fruits at every meal. For snacks, eat small amounts (1.5 ounces or a small handful) of unsalted nuts such as almonds, cashews, walnuts, and pistachios—all associated with heart health. Go easy (or eliminate altogether) protein sources that are heavy in saturated fats, such as red meat and dairy.

1. Air-Fried Spicy Chinese Eggplant

Ingredients:

1 pound Asian eggplant

1 tbsp kosher salt

2 tbsp oil

1/2 pound ground turkey

2 tsp soy sauce

2 tbsp Chinese rice wine

1 tbsp garlic, minced

1 tsp ginger, skin removed, minced

1/2 tsp Szechuan peppercorns, crushed

1 tbsp Chinese chili paste

2 tsp sugar

2 tbsp Chinese black vinegar

1 tsp cornstarch

1/2 tsp sesame oil

1 scallion, chopped

Directions for the eggplant:

Trim tops off eggplant. Cut eggplant into ¾-inch thick pieces, about 3 inches in length.

Place in a bowl. Cover with cold water and 1 tbsp kosher salt. Let sit for 15 minutes.

Drain eggplant, rinse under cold water, and pat dry with paper towels.

Return eggplant to a dry bowl. Toss with one tbsp oil.

Air Fry eggplant at 390-400 degrees for about 15 minutes, until the inside flesh is tender.

For the sauce:

While eggplant is air-frying, prepare the Eggplant Meat Sauce.

Marinate ground turkey with soy sauce and 1 tsp rice wine for 15 minutes.

Heat 1 tbsp oil in a wok or large skillet.

Add garlic and ginger: Stir-fry until fragrant, about 30 seconds. Add crushed Szechuan peppercorns and chili paste. Cook for another minute.

Add marinated meat and stir-fry until brown.

Add rice wine, sugar, vinegar, and 3 tbsp water. Bring to a boil; then reduce heat and add air-fried eggplant. Toss and simmer for 2-3 minutes.

Mix cornstarch with 2 tsp cold water. Stir into eggplant to thicken sauce.

Drizzle with sesame oil and toss. Garnish with chopped scallions.

2. Vegan Enchiladas With Lentils and Sweet Potato

Ingredients:

Sauce

4 tomatoes

½ white onion

3 garlic cloves with peel

1-2 whole chile ancho

½ cup of boiling water

1 tsp salt

Filling

1 tsp vegetable oil

3 cups sweet potatoes, diced

½ chopped white onion

2 cloves garlic, chopped

1 cup cooked lentils

1 tbsp salt

Toppings

Avocado

Cilantro

Sunflower seeds or pips

12 corn tortillas

Directions:

Soak the chile ancho in boiling water and set it aside. In a non-stick pan, roast the tomatoes, onion, and garlic until charred.

When the chili is soft, add it to the blender with the tomatoes, onion, and garlic. Add the salt and blend until everything is well integrated.

To make the filling, add 1 tbsp of oil in a large pan with the garlic, onion, and sweet potato. Leave for about 10 minutes, or until the sweet potato is al dente. Add the lentils, salt, and taste for seasoning.

Preheat the oven to 350 degrees Fahrenheit.

In a baking pan, pour a half cup of sauce at the bottom of a baking dish.

Heat the tortillas to soften (you need them to be pliable). In the center of the tortilla, layer a scoop of the lentils and sweet potato mix.

Roll the tortilla and place it on the baking dish with the seam side down.

Top the enchiladas with the remaining sauce.

Bake for 20 minutes.

Serve the enchiladas with cilantro, avocado slices, and sunflower seeds.

3. Keto Broccoli Cheese Soup

Ingredients:

1 tbsp butter

1/2 large onion, chopped

2 cloves garlic, minced

3 cups chicken broth

1 1/2 cups heavy cream

4 cups broccoli, finely chopped

1/2 tsp smoked paprika

1 tsp pepper

1/2 tsp salt

3 1/2 cups cheddar cheese

Directions:

In a deep pot, add the butter and place it over medium heat. Once hot, add the onions and garlic and stir fry for 1-2 minutes, until fragrant. Add the chicken broth, heavy cream, finely chopped broccoli, smoked paprika, pepper, and salt, and bring it to a boil. Once it begins to boil, reduce to low and simmer for 20 minutes until the broccoli is tender.

Add the cheddar cheese, half a cup at a time, until combined. Remove from the heat and serve with extra shredded cheese and chopped parsley on top.

4. Crock Pot Cauliflower Chicken Chili

Ingredients for the chili:

½ head cauliflower, diced

1 onion, diced

1 red bell pepper, diced

1 poblano pepper, diced

2 garlic cloves, minced

1 28- ounce can organic tomato puree

½ cup chicken stock

2 tbsp chili powder

¼ - ½ tsp chipotle chile flakes

1 tsp sea salt

½ tsp freshly ground pepper

6 boneless skinless chicken thighs, cut in large

chunks

Lime

Avocado

Cilantro

Directions:

Add all chili ingredients to a crock pot and stir to combine.

Cook on low for 8 hours. Taste and adjust seasonings.

Cube avocado, cut lime into wedges, and chop fresh cilantro.

Serve chili topped with avocado, a squeeze of lime juice, and cilantro to taste.

5. Sriracha Chicken Lettuce Wraps

Ingredients:

1 tbsp avocado oil

1/2 onion, diced

1½ lb skinless boneless chicken thighs, cut into bite-sized pieces

3 garlic cloves, minced

1 cup chopped celery

1 carrot, shredded

3 tbsp sugar-free sriracha sauce

3 tbsp coconut aminos

2 tbsp honey

12 leaves of bibb, butter, or romaine lettuce

Sesame seeds and chopped green onions for garnish

Directions:

Heat oil in a large skillet over medium high heat.

Add onion and sauté for 3 minutes.

Add chicken and cook, stirring for about 10 minutes, until browned on all sides.

Stir in garlic, celery, and carrots, and cook for 3 minutes.

Pour in sriracha, coconut aminos, and honey, and stir until the sauce is thickened and the chicken is coated.

Remove from heat and garnish with sesame seeds and green onions.

Serve in lettuce leaves.

6. Slow Cooker Seafood Ramen

Ingredients:

64 oz broth (seafood, vegetable, or chicken

4–6 oz ramen

1 lb seafood

2 green onions, sliced

2 tbsp low-sodium soy sauce

2 tbsp rice vinegar

2 garlic cloves, minced

1/4 cup kale, chopped

1/2 lb tomatoes, sliced

1/4 tsp sesame oil

1 tsp salt

1/4 tsp pepper

1/8 tsp red pepper flakes

Directions:

Add all ingredients except the seafood, kale and ramen to the slow cooker. Stir to mix well.

Cook on high for 2-3 hours, or low for 4-6 hours.

Add seafood, kale & ramen and cook for an additional 15-30 minutes.

7. Turkey Carrot Mushroom Dumplings

Ingredients:

3/4 c. carrots finely julienned

1 lb ground turkey

1/2 c. mushrooms finely chopped

2 tsp soy sauce

1 tsp rice wine

1 tsp sesame oil

1/2 tsp onion powder

1/8 tsp salt

2 tsp cornstarch

30 dumpling wrappers

Directions:

Put carrots in a microwavable bowl and cover with water. Cook until tender, about 3 minutes depending on how finely shredded the carrots are. Drain and let cool.

In a large bowl, mix together cooked carrots, turkey, mushrooms, soy sauce, rice wine, sesame oil, onion powder, salt and cornstarch. Stir together until well combined.

Spoon a well rounded teaspoon of filling onto a dumpling wrapper. Seal filling with wrapper. Wrap remaining dumplings.

Bring water to boil in the bottom of the steamer pot. Place dumplings in a parchment paper lined steamer. Steam 15 minutes until cooked through.

8. Slow Grilled Chinese Char Siu Chicken

Ingredients:

1/4 c. organic brown sugar

1/4 c. raw honey

1/4 c. organic ketchup

1/4 c. gluten-free soy sauce

3 Tbsp beet powder

2 Tbsp rice vinegar

1 Tbsp gluten-free hoisin sauce

1/2 tsp Chinese five-spice powder

Sea salt and freshly ground black pepper to taste

2 1/2 lbs boneless skinless chicken thighs

Cooking oil spray

Directions:

In a large bowl, mix together brown sugar, honey, ketchup, soy sauce, beet powder, vinegar, hoisin sauce, five-spice powder, salt and pepper.

Add chicken and toss well, coating all the pieces well; cover and refrigerate for two days to marinate.

Heat grill; spray cooking oil on grates; grill chicken until cooked through, about 10 minutes per side.

9. Creamy Kabocha Squash and Roasted Red Pepper Pasta

Ingredients:

1/2 c. raw cashews

1 small kabocha squash

1 head of garlic

1/3 cauliflower, cut into large florets

1/2 medium onion (roughly chopped)

1 stalk celery, roughly chopped

1 medium carrot, roughly chopped

1/4 c. roasted red peppers, drained

2 Tbsp nutritional yeast

Optional: A pinch red pepper flakes

2 to 3 c. vegetable broth (or as needed)

Salt and black pepper, to taste

1/2 to 3/4 c. fresh basil (unpacked), sliced

2 lb gluten-free spaghetti noodles (or pasta of your choice)

Serve with:

Vegan parmesan cheese (optional)

Fresh basil, sliced

Black pepper

Directions:

Soak the cashews in water overnight. If you do not have time to, you can also bring a small pot of water to a boil, remove it from heat and add in the cashews. Allow them to soak until you blend the sauce together (which will be about 1 hour).

Preheat the oven to 400°F and position the rack to the middle of the oven. Line a baking sheet with parchment paper or a silicone mat. Wash and dry the kabocha squash, place it (whole) on the baking sheet and into the oven for 18-20 minutes. Remove the pan from the oven and cool until the squash is easy to handle. If the stem of it is protruding, use a knife to carefully remove it. Slice the squash in half vertically, then scoop out the seeds and fiber using a spoon. Slice the squash into 1-inch wedges, trying to keep the slices uniform for even cooking. Place 6 or 7 the slices of the cooked s▯uash (roughly 1 1/2 cups) onto your lined baking sheet. The remaining kabocha s▯uash can be cooked on an additional baking sheet with the same baking time and directions below. It can be stored in the fridge in an airtight container for up to a week.

Using your hands, remove loose skin from the outside of the head of garlic. With a sharp knife, cut 1/4"-inch off the top of the garlic, or enough to expose the tops of the cloves. Place the garlic head (cut side down) onto the baking sheet along with the cauliflower florets, onions, celery, and carrots. Sprinkle with salt and pepper and place back into the oven for 40 minutes, flipping/mixing halfway through.

10 minutes before the vegetables are done, prepare the pasta.

Once you have removed the baking sheet from the oven, allow the veggies to cool until easily handled and then use a knife to carefully remove the skin from the kabocha and add it into a high speed blender. You can discard this or snack on it as you continue cooking. Using you hands, squeeze the soften garlic cloves out of the head and into the blender, along with the soaked cashews (drained), the remaining vegetables on the baking sheet, the roasted red peppers, nutritional yeast, red pepper flakes, 2 cups of vegetable broth plus salt and pepper as desired. Blend until smooth, adding as much of the additional 1 cup of vegetable broth as needed to thin out the sauce. Adjust seasonings to taste and then add in the sliced basil. Pulse the basil in until well combined (do not blend it as it will turn the sauce a weird color).

Drain the pasta, add it back into the pot and pour over the sauce. Mix until well combined.

Serve with a sprinkle of fresh parmesan, basil and black pepper. Enjoy!

10. Loaded Cauliflower

Ingredients:

1.25 lb cauliflower head, cut into florets

6 green onion, chopped into the green and white parts

2 tbsp butter

3 garlic cloves, minced

2 oz cream cheese

1/2 tsp sea salt

1/4 tsp black pepper

1.5 tsp ranch seasoning Mix, optional

3/4 c. organic heavy whipping cream

2 c. cheddar cheese, grated

4 slices sugar-free bacon, crumbled

Olive oil for roasting the cauliflower

Dollops of sour cream, optional

Directions:

Preheat the oven to 425 degrees.

Toss the cauliflower with ~2 Tbsp of olive oil then add it to a baking sheet. Roast the cauliflower on a baking sheet for 25 minutes. The cauliflower will get tender and some parts will brown up.

While the cauliflower is roasting, make the cheese sauce: Add butter, the white parts of the green onions, and the garlic cloves to a skillet on medium heat. Sauté until the onions are translucent (~3 minutes).

Add heavy cream, cream cheese, salt, ranch seasoning (if you're using it), and pepper to the skillet with the onions, garlic and butter. Turn the heat to medium low and continue to cook until the cream cheese is melted. Stir in 1.5

cups of the cheddar cheese to finish the cheese sauce.

Mix the cheese sauce and the roasted cauliflower, then add it to a baking dish. Top it with the remaining cheddar cheese and roast for an additional 20 minutes, or until the cauliflower is tender.

Top the baked cauliflower, with some dollops of sour cream, the green parts of the green onions, and the crumbled bacon.

11. Easy Creamy Cajun Shrimp Pasta

Ingredients:

8 oz linguine pasta

2 tsp olive oil Divided into 1 teaspoon servings.

1 lb raw shrimp, deveined and shells removed.

1 Tbsp cajun seasoning divided into 1/2 Tbsp servings. You can also use creole seasoning.

4 oz andouille sausage Sliced into 1 inch pieces.

You can use more if you like.

1/2 c. chopped red peppers

1/2 c. chopped green peppers

1/2 c. chopped yellow or white onions

1 c. fire roasted diced tomatoes Drained from a

can.

1 Tbsp butter

1/2 c. heavy whipping cream

1/2 c. unsweetened almond milk

4 oz cream cheese Cut into chunks.

1/2 c. shredded Parmesan Reggiano Cheese

Directions:

Cook the pasta as per package instructions.

Place the shrimp in a bowl along with 1/2 Tbsp

of cajun or creole seasoning. Mix to ensure the

shrimp is fully coated.

Heat a skillet or pan on medium high heat. I use a cast iron skillet. Add 1 teaspoon of olive oil to the pan.

When hot, add the shrimp to the pan. Cook for 2-3 minutes on each side until it turns bright pink. Remove the shrimp and set aside.

Add an additional teaspoon of olive oil to the pan along with the chopped sausage, onions, green peppers, and red peppers.

Saute for 3-4 minutes until the vegetables are soft and the onions are translucent and fragrant. Remove the vegetables from the pan and set aside.

Reduce the heat on the pan to medium. Add the butter to the pan and allow it to melt.

Add in the heavy cream, almond milk, cream cheese, the remaining 1/2 tablespoon of cajun or creole seasoning, and parmesan reggiano cheese.

Continue to stir the sauce until all of the cheese has fully melted. The cream cheese may take some time to melt. Add in the fire roasted tomatoes and stir. Allow the mixture to cook for 2 minutes.

Add the shrimp, sausage, vegetables, and pasta to the pan and stir. Allow the pasta to cook for 4-5 minutes until combined. Serve.

12. Healthy Chicken Taco Soup

Ingredients:

½ Tbsp avocado or coconut oil

1 small yellow onion, diced

1 small red bell pepper, diced

1 small green bell pepper, diced

5 cloves garlic, minced

1 lb boneless, skinless chicken breast

1 1/2 tsp salt (plus more to taste)

1 tsp dried oregano

1 tsp chipotle powder

1 tsp paprika

2 tsp cumin

¼ tsp black pepper

1 – 15 oz can fire roasted diced tomatoes

2 – 4.5 oz cans green chilies

¼ c. fresh lime juice

32 oz chicken broth

Cilantro, for serving

Diced red onion, for serving

Lime wedges, for serving

Directions:

Heat a large pot over medium-high heat. Once
hot, add in the avocado or coconut oil. Next,
add the peppers, onion, and garlic to the pot.
Saute for 3-4 minutes until the onions start to
become translucent.

Add the chicken breast, canned tomatoes, canned green chilies, spices, lime juice, and chicken broth to the pot. Stir until well combined. Bring the soup to a rolling boil and then reduce the heat to a simmer. Allow the soup to simmer for 30 minutes or until the chicken is tender and easy to shred.

Transfer the chicken breast from the soup to a small bowl. Use two forks to shred the meat. Add the chicken back to the soup and stir until well combined. Serve the soup with fresh cilantro, diced red onion, and fresh lime wedges. Enjoy!

13. Quick and Easy Mongolian Beef

Ingredients:

1 lb flank steak thinly sliced against the grain

2 Tbsp cornstarch

2-4 Tbsp canola oil

1 yellow onion sliced

2 green onions chopped, green and white parts
separated

4 garlic cloves chopped

1- inch ginger chopped

¼ c. low sodium soy sauce

¼ c. water

1 Tbsp hoisin sauce

3 Tbsp brown sugar

Salt to taste

Directions:

Cover the flank steak with cornstarch, making
sure each piece is covered. Set aside.

Heat the canola oil in a large skillet over
medium-high heat. Once the oil is hot, add the
flank steak to the frying pan in a single layer,
making sure that the pieces are not touching.

Cook for 1-2 minutes per side until each side is browned. Cook in batches until all the flank steak is cooked. Set aside.

Add sliced yellow onion, whites of green onions, garlic, and ginger to the skillet and stir fry for about 3 minutes, until the onions are slightly softened but still have a little crunch. Add soy sauce, water, hoisin sauce, and brown sugar and stir. Add steak back to the pan along with the green parts of the onions. Remove from heat and serve.

14. Caribbean Steamed Fish

Ingredients:

2 lbs fish (porgy or snapper), cleaned and scaled

Juice of 1 lime

½ tsp black pepper

1 tsp salt

3 cloves garlic – 2 sliced and 1 crushed

About 15 sprigs thyme

½ Tbsp butter

½ Tbsp oil

2 carrots, thinly sliced

1 red pepper, thinly sliced

1 green pepper, thinly sliced

1 onion, thinly sliced

12 okra, ends cut off

1 hot pepper (scotch bonnet, habanero or wiri wiri), seeds removed

1 ½ cup water

Directions:

Season the fish with lime juice, crushed garlic, black pepper, salt and half of the thyme and set aside.

In a large, wide heavy bottom pot over medium heat, add oil and butter. When butter has melted, sauté carrots, red and green pepper, and onion until it has softened, about 5 minutes.

Add garlic slices and pepper and cook for just a minute or two. Add water and bring to a boil. Add fish to the pot. Spoon some of the vegetables on top of the fish. Add okra and the rest of the thyme.

Cover the pot and lower the heat to simmer then cook for 15 minutes until the fish is done. Remove from heat and serve.

15. Corn Chowder Con Chile Poblano

Ingredients:

2 Tbsp vegetable oil

1 poblano pepper without seeds and thinly sliced

1 medium onion sliced

2 cloves of garlic roughly chopped

5 corn husks

4 medium potatoes cubed

1 tsp of salt

To serve:

Corn kernels

Pumpkin seeds

Cilantro microgreens or chopped cilantro

Olive oil

Freshly ground pepper

Directions:

In a large pot add the oil and the sliced poblano chile. Leave it there until it begins to soften. Add the onion and garlic. Leave for five more minutes or until you see that the onion is translucent.

Add the corn kernels, potatoes, salt and cover with water, add the salt and cover. Leave for 10-15 minutes or until the vegetables are cooked.

With a ladle, add about one-third of the vegetables and liquid into the container of a blender. Blend until fully liquefied and well integrated. Return to the pot with the rest of the vegetables. If you need more liquid, add a little more water. Check for seasoning and adjust if necessary.

Serve with a drizzle of olive oil, pumpkin seeds, corn kernels, sprouts or chopped cilantro. Finish with sea salt and pepper.

16. Crispy Potato Tacos

Ingredients:

12 corn tortillas

1 c. mashed potatoes

4 Tbsp of vegetable oil or avocado oil

4 long wooden skewers

To serve:

Thinly sliced romaine lettuce or green cabbage

Radishes thinly sliced

Cilantro

Guacamole

Salsa verde

Directions:

Heat tortillas on a skillet for 10-15 seconds to make them pliable.

Put a spoonful of mashed potatoes in the center of each tortilla and spread it along the tortilla. Roll the tortilla and put it on a long skewer. Repeat until you put three or four tacos on the skewer.

Repeat with all the tortillas.

In a frying pan over high heat put a tablespoon of oil and put three or four tacos, leave until golden brown, three to five minutes, turn and brown on the other side.

Take out the tacos and put in a dish with a paper towel to absorb the excess oil.

Repeat until all the tacos are done.

To serve, put the crispy potato tacos on a plate and finish with the toppings. Enjoy immediately.

17. Black Garlic, Sesame, and Shitake Cod

Ingredients:

2 Alaskan Cod filets, frozen

1 clove black garlic

2 Tbsp olive oil

1 tsp sesame seeds

1/2 c. dried shiitake, rehydrated

Directions:

Preheat your oven to 450F.

Rinse frozen fish, pat dry with a paper towel, and place on a non-stick pan.

In a small bowl, place black garlic and warm in the microwave for 10 seconds.

Mash the garlic clove and add olive oil and sesame seeds.

Brush this mixture on frozen filets and sprinkle the mushrooms around the fish.

Place in the oven for 12-15 minutes, depending on the thickness of the fish. If your filets are on the thick side, flip halfway through cooking.

Serve alongside rice, your favorite salad, or whole grain.

18. Shrimp Lettuce Wraps

Ingredients:

1 head butter lettuce or romaine lettuce hearts

¼ c. low-sodium chicken broth

1 Tbsp hoisin sauce

½ Tbsp low-sodium soy sauce

1 tsp rice vinegar

¼ tsp Asian sesame oil

1 1/2 tsp chili garlic sauce

½ tsp cornstarch

1 Tbsp canola or avocado oil divided

30 grams cashews little less than ¼ cup, coarsely chopped

6 oz shrimp deveined & cut into small cubes

1 large garlic clove minced

1/2 large red bell pepper seeded and diced

3 green onions the white and green parts, sliced

⅛ c. chopped cilantro

1 carrot shredded or cut into thin strips

Directions:

Divide the lettuce into leaves and set aside.

In a small bowl, whisk together the chicken broth, hoisin sauce, soy sauce, rice vinegar, sesame oil, chili garlic sauce, and cornstarch. Set aside.

In a medium skillet, heat ½ Tbsp canola or avocado oil over medium-high heat until almost smoking.

Add the shrimp and stir-fry until browned. About 2 minutes. Transfer the shrimp to a plate and discard any juices from the pan.

In the same skillet, heat the other ½ tablespoon of oil over medium-high heat.

Add the garlic, bell pepper, green onions, and carrots.

Stir fry until tender-crisp, about 2 minutes.

Return the shrimp to the pan and add the cashews and cilantro. Add the soy-sauce mixture and stir-fry until the shrimp is thoroughly cooked. About 3 minutes.

Spoon the shrimp mixture evenly onto lettuce leaves.

19. Baked Salmon Cake Balls With Rosemary Aioli

Ingredients:

2 lbs wild salmon fillets

1 tsp sea salt

1 tsp black pepper

1/2 medium purple onion, chopped

1/2 c. organic spinach, chopped

1/2 red bell pepper, diced

1/2 yellow red pepper, diced

1 small jalapeño, diced

2/3 c. breadcrumbs

1-2 Tbsps Old Bay seasoning

1/2 c. fresh parsley, chopped

1/3 c. vegan Mayo

1/2 c. dijon mustard

1 large organic egg, room temp.

4 Tbsps lemon juice

1-2 Tbsps sriracha sauce

1/2 c. vegan mayo

4 tsp lemon juice

2 garlic cloves, crushed + minced

1/4 tsp sea salt

2 sprigs fresh rosemary, chopped

Directions:

First, preheat the oven to 400 degrees Fahrenheit.

Season salmon with sea salt + black pepper and roast on a baking sheet (lined with parchment paper) for about 20 minutes, or until cooked through.

Once cooked, remove from the oven and set aside while it cools for 5 minutes before shredding or flaking into medium chunks.

Meanwhile, add onions, bell peppers, jalapeños, spinach, old bay seasoning, breadcrumbs, parsley, mayo, dijon mustard, egg, sriracha and lemon juice to a large bowl. Then add shredded salmon and mix all ingredients together, using your hands.

Scoop about 2 Tbsps of batter and form into a ball with your hands and line on a baking sheet (lined with parchment paper). Repeat until all batter is used.

Bake salmon balls for 15-20 minutes, or until slightly crisp and golden brown.

Combine vegan mayo, lemon juice, garlic cloves, sea salt, and rosemary in a medium bowl and whisk together thoroughly. Refrigerate for aioli until ready to use.